TEEN MENTAL HEALTH™

gender identity

Nicki Peter Petrikowski

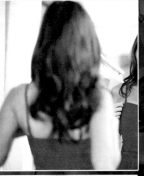

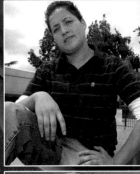

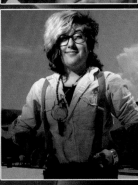

ROSEN
PUBLISHING

New York

305.3
P

Published in 2014 by The Rosen Publishing Group, Inc.
29 East 21st Street, New York, NY 10010

First Edition

Library of Congress Cataloging-in-Publication Data

Petrikowski, Nicki Peter.
Gender identity/Nicki Peter Petrikowski.–First edition.
    pages cm.–(Teen mental health)
Includes bibliographical references and index.
ISBN 978-1-4777-1748-6 (library binding)
1. Transgender people–Popular works. 2. Gender identity–Popular works. 3. Adolescent psychology–Popular works. I. Title.
HQ77.9.P48 2014
305.3–dc23

2013012069

Manufactured in the United States of America

CPSIA Compliance Information: Batch #W14YA: For further information, contact Rosen Publishing, New York, New York, at 1-800-237-9932.

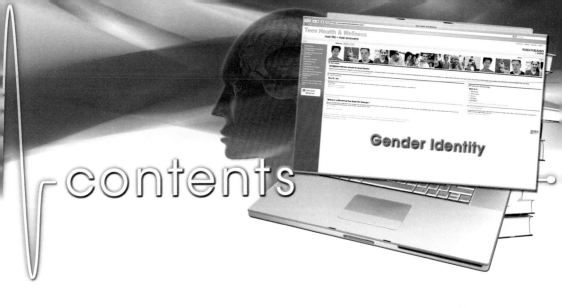

contents

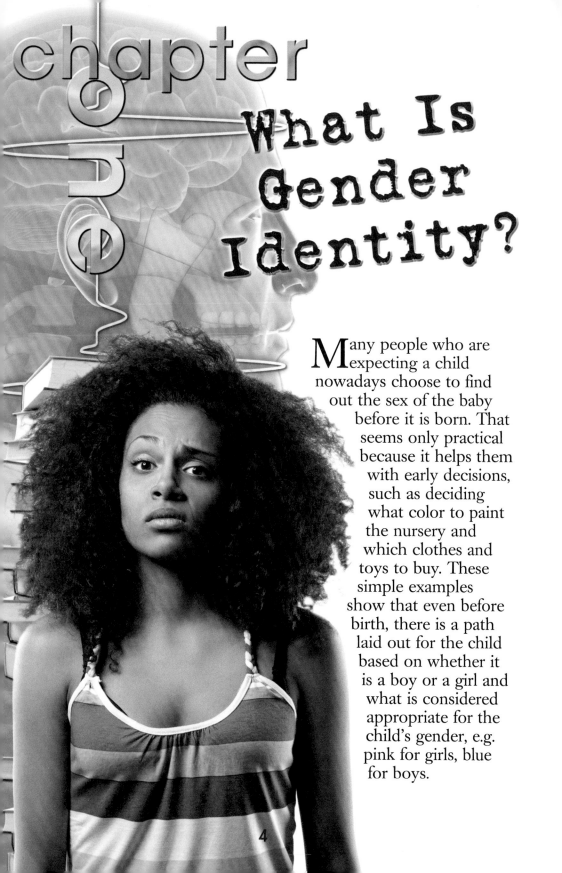

chapter one

What Is Gender Identity?

Many people who are expecting a child nowadays choose to find out the sex of the baby before it is born. That seems only practical because it helps them with early decisions, such as deciding what color to paint the nursery and which clothes and toys to buy. These simple examples show that even before birth, there is a path laid out for the child based on whether it is a boy or a girl and what is considered appropriate for the child's gender, e.g. pink for girls, blue for boys.

For most people, making purchases based on gender is not a problem, and they don't ever question it because it suits their own life without any complications. But for some, the matter is not as clear-cut. For them, what is expected of their gender does not feel right. This can range from a girl who would rather play with model cars (or another toy that is generally thought of as being for boys) instead of dolls to a boy feeling more comfortable in girls' clothing to people believing that they were born in the wrong body.

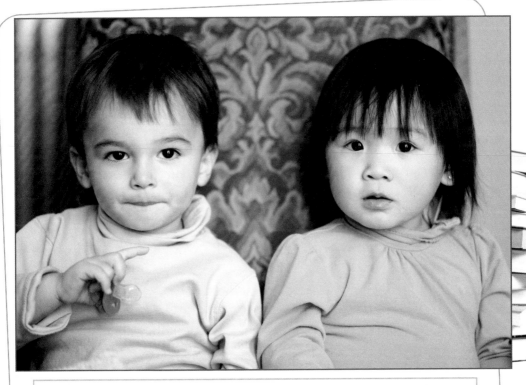

Many decisions are made for children depending on their sex. The typical color of their clothes is just one obvious example of this.

The Difference Between Sex and Gender

To understand what is meant by gender identity, it is important to first understand the distinction between sex and gender. Although these terms are often thought to be interchangeable, that is incorrect. There are several physical attributes that determine if a person is anatomically male or female, their biological sex. These attributes include chromosomes, gonads, hormones, and the internal and external reproductive organs. A newborn baby is assigned a sex at birth based on these physical attributes.

Gender is a concept that is not directly based on those physical attributes but on what society associates with and expects from those who have those attributes. There is no real reason why the nursery for a girl will often be painted pink and for a boy will be painted blue. The only reason is that those colors are commonly associated with the respective genders, and children are expected to like the color associated with their gender. This means they will learn from an early age what is considered appropriate for them based on the reactions they get in regard to not only colors, but also clothes, toys, sports, and countless other things. For example, many males are told while growing up that boys don't cry, while for girls, it is socially acceptable to cry. Men and women, boys and girls, are expected to behave a certain way. How much they are in line with the gender roles formed by the society they live in has an influence on how they are perceived by others.

Gender is a social construct. That means in different societies (in different countries, but also in different groups within the same country), there can be differences between what is thought of as masculine or feminine, what is considered appropriate for a man or woman. For example, many Americans would find it strange to see a man wearing a

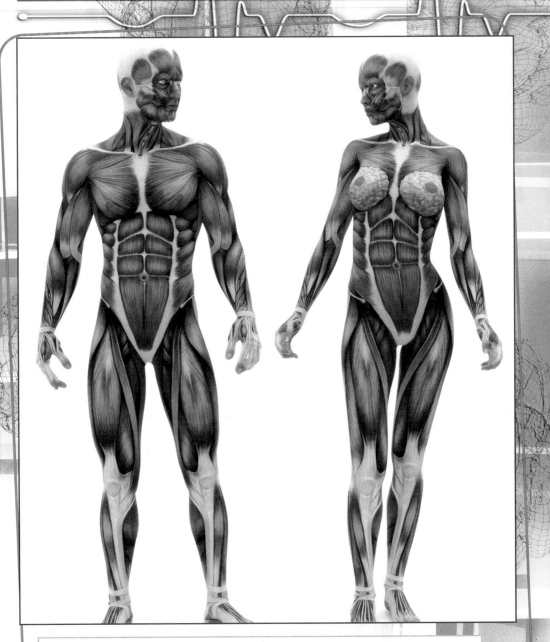

Certain anatomical features determine the biological sex of a human's body, but they do not determine a person's gender identity.

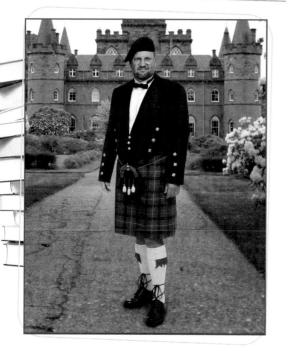

What kind of clothes are deemed appropriate for a man or a woman can differ from country to country, as this Scotsman's traditional attire shows.

skirt. But in Scotland, nobody would be taken aback by a man in a kilt.

It is worth keeping in mind that these gender roles are not set in stone; they can and frequently do change. What is expected from and considered appropriate for men and women today is different from what it was even a generation or two ago. Most likely, it will be different in the future.

Gender Identity and Gender Expression

One aspect that is ingrained very deeply in society is the belief that there are only two genders, male and female. This belief is referred to as gender binary. In this belief system, it is expected that people's behavior will correspond to their anatomy. A person who is biologically male is supposed to be masculine, while a person who is biologically female is supposed to be feminine.

It is becoming ever apparent that the world is not as simple as that concept, and society is slowly accepting that fact. It is more important not to think of gender as a binary system with two clear opposites, one of which any given person has to belong to. Instead, gender should be thought of as a spectrum. Every person has a gender identity, an internal sense of being a boy or a girl, a man

MYTHS AND FACTS

Myth: Young people don't yet know their gender identity.

Fact: According to Stephanie Brill and Rachel Pepper's book *The Transgender Child*, "gender identity emerges around the same time as a child learns to speak." So some children tell their parents at a very young age that they are transgender, but they are not always taken seriously when the parents dismiss it as a phase that will pass. Other people may know that something is not quite right but can't figure it out until years later, sometimes well into adulthood. In some cases, it takes the professional help of a psychiatrist for people to realize that they are transgender.

Myth: It is a choice to be transgender.

Fact: While we do not know at this point what exactly makes a person transgender, it is understood to be a biological reason, whether it is genetics or the exposure to hormones or environmental factors. For transgender people, it is not a choice—they were born that way. Their only choice would be to suppress what they know about themselves, which is not healthy.

Myth: All transgender people are gay.

Fact: There is a difference between gender identity and sexual orientation. The inner sense of one's gender does not say anything about who one is romantically and sexually attracted to. Like non-transgender people, transgender people can be attracted to a person of the same or different gender—or both or none at all. Some transgender people are gay, and others are heterosexual.

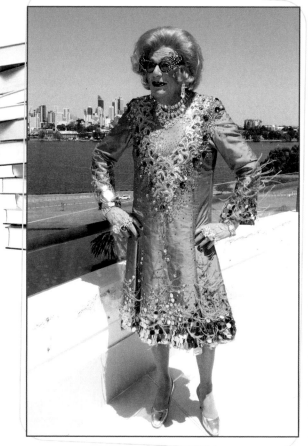

Dame Edna Everage, a character Australian comedian Barry Humphries has been performing as for decades, is famous for her flamboyant gender expression.

or a woman, or maybe neither of the two or a bit of both. That is where the gender binary proves to be too restrictive.

Gender expression is the way that someone shows gender externally, through movement, mannerisms and speech, but also through signals like clothing and hairstyles. In many cases, these are not conscious decisions, but they can be. How people express themselves is what we notice and often base assumptions on. However, it is important to remember that people's gender expression does not necessarily tell something about their gender identity or their sex. For example, a short-haired woman wearing a suit might easily be mistaken for a man, while her appearance allows no conclusion to be drawn about her gender identity, which is something only she could tell you.

People whose gender identity and/or gender expression does not line up with their anatomical sex can be referred to as gender nonconforming or transgender.

(The Latin word *trans* means "across." Transgender people go across what are traditionally considered gender boundaries.)

Contrary to the concept of gender binary, gender as a spectrum does not offer clear-cut categories in which one can easily fit people. This is because the relationship between sex, gender identity, and gender expression varies from individual to individual. Nonetheless, the next section will take a look at different forms of being transgender. It is worth keeping in mind that there is little black and white and a lot of grey areas where transgenderism is concerned.

Where it can get a little confusing is when people first come out as gay or lesbian and later realize that they are transsexual, which means they are not actually homosexual as they originally thought because they are in fact attracted to people of a different gender. It is also possible that people in a heterosexual relationship, even a marriage, can discover that they are transsexual. In this case the partners have to figure out where they stand on an individual basis. Some couples decide to split up, while others stay together because they love one another, despite never thinking themselves to be homosexual.

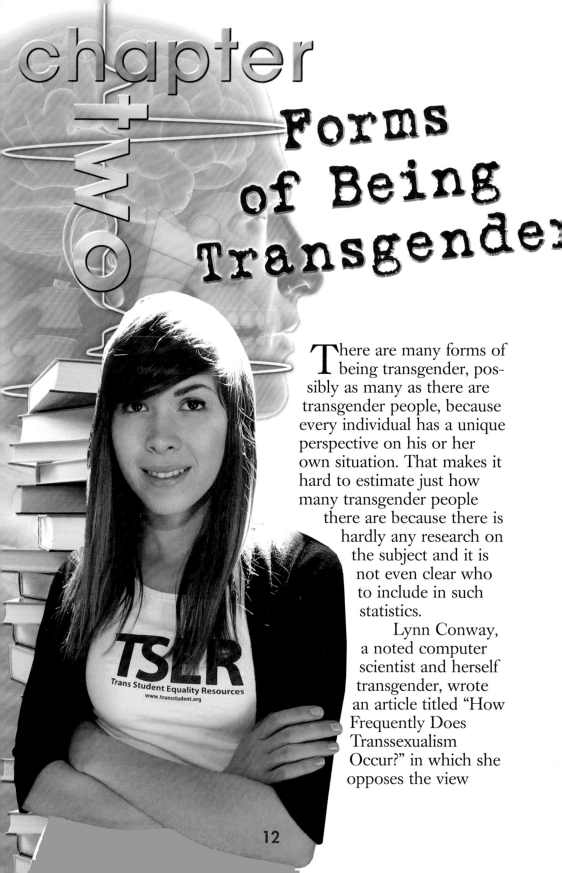

chapter two

Forms of Being Transgender

There are many forms of being transgender, possibly as many as there are transgender people, because every individual has a unique perspective on his or her own situation. That makes it hard to estimate just how many transgender people there are because there is hardly any research on the subject and it is not even clear who to include in such statistics.

Lynn Conway, a noted computer scientist and herself transgender, wrote an article titled "How Frequently Does Transsexualism Occur?" in which she opposes the view based on decades-old statistics that one in thirty thousand males is a male-to-female transsexual. She estimates that the number may be one in five hundred or even higher. That does not include other forms of being transgender, which make it an even more common phenomenon.

While it is unknown at this point how many transgender people there are, the number apparently is higher than many have believed. It might be a comfort for transgender people to know that they are not alone.

Transsexuals

Transsexuals are people who do not identify with the sex they were assigned at birth and who strive to live permanently as the gender they do identify with. Often they not only dress accordingly but also change their bodies hormonally or surgically, as they want their physical sex to conform to their internal sense of gender identity.

A transsexual person labeled at birth as male but who identifies as female is called a transgirl/transwoman, or MTF/M2F (male-to-female transperson). A transsexual person labeled at birth as female but who identifies as male is called a transboy/transman, or FTM/F2M (female-to-male transperson). Many people are not aware that transmen exist, but it is a myth that there are only MTF transsexuals. The explanation for the general perception being wrong in this case might be that transwomen tend to be more noticeable due to physical characteristics, such as their height or prominent jawline.

Not only would it be rude to say that a transwoman is not really a woman or a transboy is actually a girl, it is also incorrect based on the distinction between sex and gender. Transgender people should be treated like the gender they present themselves as, which includes using the name they have chosen for themselves, as well

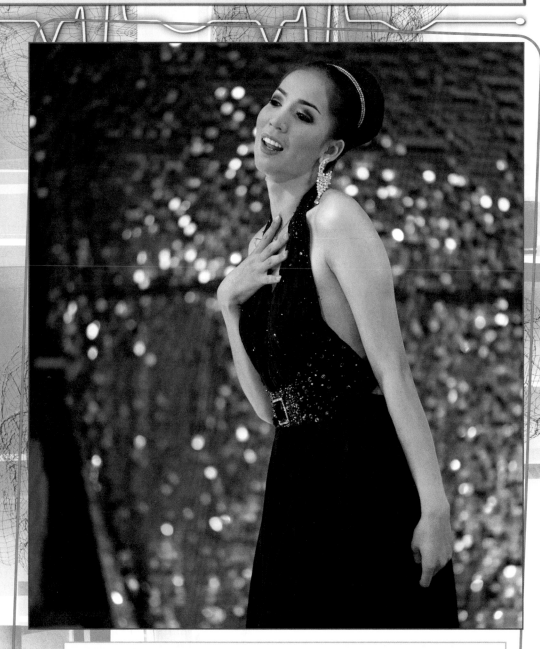

This transsexual singer shows that it can be difficult, if not impossible, to tell when people present themselves as a gender that is different than their sex.

as the appropriate pronoun. A transgirl/transwoman should be called "she," and a transboy/trasman "he." However, some transgender people prefer the use of a gender-neutral pronoun, such as "ze" or "hir," while others avoid the use of pronouns altogether and prefer their name to be used in all cases where a pronoun would usually be used. If in doubt, it is always an option to ask respectfully how a person would like to be addressed.

Cross-dressers, Drag Queens, and Drag Kings

Cross-dressers are people who wear clothes and/or accessories that are generally thought of as being reserved for the opposite gender. Cross-dressers can be male-to-female or female-to-male, although women in men's clothing are probably less noticeable and more socially accepted than men in women's clothing. While there are some who derive sexual pleasure from their cross-dressing, others do not and cross-dress simply because it makes them feel comfortable.

Unlike transsexuals, cross-dressers usually identify with the sex they were assigned at birth and do not seek to transition and live permanently as the opposite sex, which can lead to some tension between the two groups, as some cross-dressers think transsexuals are taking things too far, while some transsexuals think that cross-dressers are not taking things far enough. Cross-dressers also used to be called transvestites, but that is now considered a negative term and should not be used.

Drag queens and drag kings differ from cross-dressers in that they dress as the opposite gender for the purpose of entertaining (singing, dancing etc.), rather than for their own well-being. Drag queens are men who dress and perform as women, and drag kings are women who dress and perform as men while often exaggerating certain characteristics. Drag

15

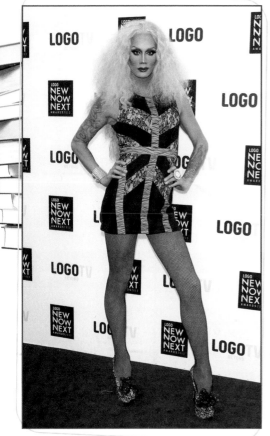

The popularity of drag performers such as Raja makes it clear that this form of entertainment is entering the mainstream, raising awareness of issues of gender identity.

was and still is popular in the gay community, but all performers are not necessarily gay and one does not need to be gay to enjoy it.

Genderqueer

"Genderqueer" is a term growing in popularity. It refers to people who feel that they are neither completely male nor female but in between. Sometimes people who identify as genderqueer will later seek full transition, but others accept their gender as genderqueer permanently and live their lives accordingly. Typically, gender identity, gender expression, and sexual orientation are not static categories for genderqueer individuals. Instead these are considered changeable.

Gender Nonconforming and Gender Variant

"Gender nonconforming" is a very broad term, as strictly speaking it encompasses any behavior and interest that is not in line with the traditional notion of a given gender. Nearly every person will be gender nonconforming at one point or another, be it a husband who cooks a meal for his wife or a woman who likes to watch sports. Fortunately, these things are no longer seen as the oddities they were perceived as not long ago, showing that the concept of gender is not static. More specifically, "gender nonconforming" is a term used for those who do not conform to societal expectations on a more regular basis.

Often people do not identify themselves as gender nonconforming but are perceived as such by others. This is more often the case with boys or men engaging in stereotypically feminine behavior than the other way around. The reason for this is that there is generally more acceptance in society for a certain amount of tomboyishness, but women who express themselves in a particularly masculine manner may also be met with resentment. Gender nonconforming individuals may identify as transgender or genderqueer, but often their gender identity is in line with their birth sex. They may also be lesbian, gay, or bisexual. However, all gender nonconforming people are not homosexual or bisexual. Likewise, all homosexual or bisexual individuals are not gender nonconforming. "Gender nonconforming" and "gender variant" can mean the same thing. However, some people make a distinction between the two based on how the individual in question is perceived by others.

Tomboys are girls who express themselves in ways that are typically associated with boys, such as clothing style and preferred hobbies.

17

Intersex

The Intersex Society of North America (ISNA) defines intersex as "a general term used for a variety of conditions in which a person is born with a reproductive or sexual anatomy that doesn't seem to fit the typical definitions of female or male." An intersex person is anatomically between male and female (the Latin word *inter* means "between"), for which there are a number of different causes (including the influence of certain hormones or mutations of chromosomes or genes) that lead to different conditions. Some are so subtle that the people with these conditions may only notice them later in life or sometimes not at all. Others are obvious and can have a severe impact on the person in question because, for example, they may be infertile. According to the ISNA, the body of 1 in 100 people differs from the standard male or female form at birth; in about 1 in 1,500 to 1 in 2,000 births, the condition is so noticeable that a specialist is called in.

As the name says, intersex is a matter of anatomical sex, not of gender. For many intersex people, their gender identity corresponds to the sex they were labeled with at birth. Others may be transgender, but that does not have to be connected to their intersex condition, which, as noted, does not have to be severe and can be so subtle as to be unnoticeable.

For others, gender identity will be an issue because of their intersex condition. In the past, it was common to surgically adjust the anatomy of a child born with an intersex condition to make that child look typically male or female. The problem with this, of course, is that the doctors could make a decision that did not correspond to the child's gender identity. While this practice still exists today, it is

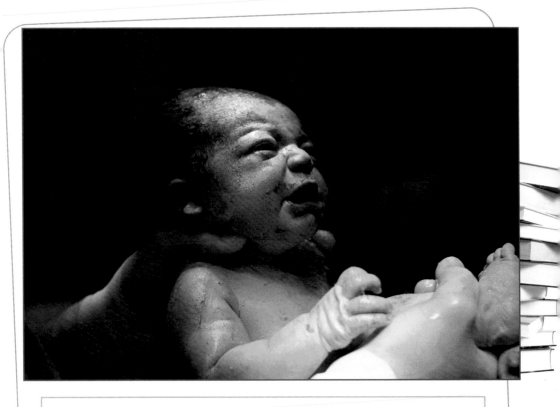

In a lot of cases, determining the sex of an intersex child at birth can cause problems down the road.

advisable to wait on such a far-reaching determination until the person affected by it can make the choice on his or her own.

Whether intersex people see themselves as transgender or consider their condition to be a purely medical one is up to them. One thing to remember is that sex, much like gender, is not the binary that many people consider it to be, but a spectrum that covers more than just the poles of male and female.

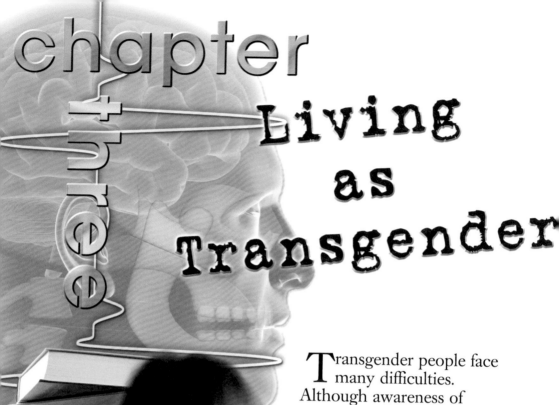

chapter three

Living as Transgender

Transgender people face many difficulties. Although awareness of transgender people is high, acceptance regrettably is not at the same level. Society is changing to be more accepting of those who do not fit into traditional gender roles, but this change is occurring slowly. Instead of waiting for it to happen, it might be worthwhile to take a proactive role.

Coming Out

Disclosing one's transgenderism is not an easy step to take. Considering the reactions one can face, it is a scary thing. On the other hand, it can be a great relief to no longer feel like you have to hide and be open about yourself.

Accepting One's Self

The first person one has to come out to is oneself. For some transgender people, this is not a problem, as they are clear about who they are from an early age and accept it. Others may know they are different from what is generally presented as the norm, but they may not be able to pinpoint why they feel that way, and it can take many years until they do. There

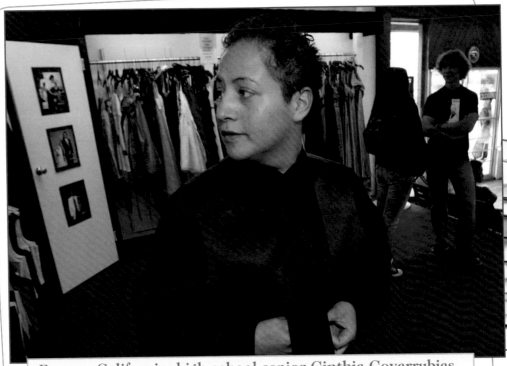

Fresno, California, high school senior Cinthia Covarrubias, the school's first transgender prom king candidate, tries on her tux. To discover who you are, you often have to take a long, hard look at yourself, and not just in the mirror.

could be confusion about whether gender identity, gender expression, or sexual orientation is the issue. Some transgender people may even suppress their feelings and hope that they will go away because they are afraid of what will happen when they admit to them.

Educating oneself is always a good idea. Another thing that can help is talking to a psychiatrist. Not all psychiatrists are knowledgeable about transgenderism, so it might be preferable to seek out a specialist. Another option is reaching out to people who have been in a similar situation and learning about their experiences. It can be very helpful and reassuring to find that you are not alone in what you are going through. Thanks to the Internet, forming and finding communities is easier than ever before. Of course, it is advisable to be cautious when dealing with strangers.

Coming Out to Others

Coming out to someone always involves a risk because not everyone is understanding; this is something that needs to be considered beforehand. It is a good idea to try to anticipate the reaction of the person whom one is coming out to and to be prepared in case that reaction is negative. It is also worth keeping in mind that the initial reaction is not necessarily the long-term one. Sometimes people need a while to come to terms with the information that they have received. In other cases, people who were understanding at first may have difficulty being accepting later on.

Compared to people coming out about their sexual orientation, it might be more difficult for transgender people to choose who they want to come out to because gender expression is visible to others while sexual orientation is not. A cross-dresser may choose to dress in the clothes usually reserved for the opposite sex only in the privacy of his or her own home, but a transsexual, genderqueer, or gender nonconforming person will in many cases be noticeable to others. That takes a lot of courage.

For most young transgender people, the first people they will come out to are their family, especially their parents. This can be difficult because not only is the parents' reaction of particular importance to a child, but also children depend on their parents in many ways. Therefore it is smart to consider beforehand what will happen should coming out to your parents mean losing their support,

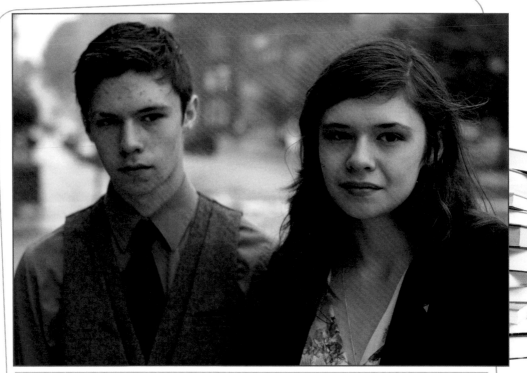

Jonas Maines (*left*) and his transgender sister, Nicole Maines, were born as identical twin boys. Coming out to others, especially to your parents, can be very difficult. However, their support can also be a great help.

emotional or otherwise. Many parents are understanding and supportive, however, because they love their child, although it might take some time for them to adjust. They may feel like they have lost their son or daughter, who they had dreams and plans for. This can be difficult for them to deal with, although their child is still the same person. Other family members and close friends may also need some time to come to terms with the person they know being different than they thought. It is a complicated process that requires patience and understanding from both sides, but it can be a rewarding experience.

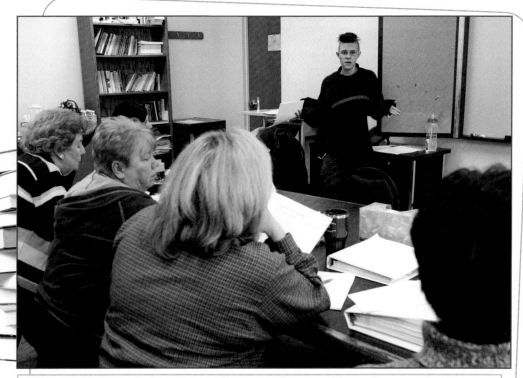

David Fischer, a twenty-year-old college student from suburban Chicago, recently started making the transition from female to male. He speaks to adults, helping them understand how to talk to transgender youth.

There are not only family and friends to think about, though. After transitioning–that is, changing from living as one gender to living as another–all people who were previously acquainted with the transgender person will notice, and word usually spreads quickly. While the opinions and reactions of these people may not matter to the transgender person as much as those of family and friends, it is still something he or she will have to deal with. Therefore some transgender people choose to move somewhere where nobody knows them after transitioning so that they can have a fresh start.

Dealing with Discrimination

Transgender people face discrimination in many aspects of life, ranging from employment to housing to health care issues, and they are frequently the targets of violence. Gender identity was added to the federal hate crimes law in 2009. The law is supposed to protect transgender people, but it only comes into play once a crime has been committed. Society as a whole has to change to be more accepting, and transgender people can do their part in bringing about this change by standing up for their cause, being role models for others, and through their efforts to make it easier for those who will follow in their footsteps.

Gender Justice in Schools

A report called "Harsh Realities" published by the Gay, Lesbian and Straight Education Network in 2009 shows that transgender students are frequently the victims of harassment and physical violence. According to the report, almost 90 percent of transgender students were verbally harassed, over half were physically harassed (e.g., pushed or shoved) and about a quarter were physically assaulted

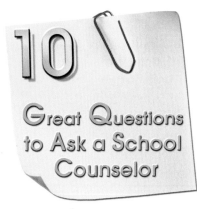

10

Great Questions to Ask a School Counselor

1. Does my school have experience with transgender issues?

2. How can I tell what my gender identity is?

3. How do I deal with coming out?

4. How can I deal with anxiety or distress as a result of coming out?

5. How can I access unbiased health care?

6. What does transitioning entail and what options are there?

7. What can I do if I feel unsafe at school?

8. How should I react to negative comments about my transgenderism?

9. Who can I go to if I'm being harassed?

10. What does my school do to prevent discrimination?

(e.g., punched or kicked) because of their sexual orientation or their gender expression over the course of the school year. Moreover, many transgender students have to deal with discrimination from the school administration. This includes being denied access to extracurricular activities, being forbidden to wear clothing that fits their gender identity, and not being referred to by their chosen name and corresponding pronoun. This behavior may not be because of malice but because of ignorance, which is something that the students and their parents can help fix.

The law protects transgender students from harassment, and schools are legally required to take steps against

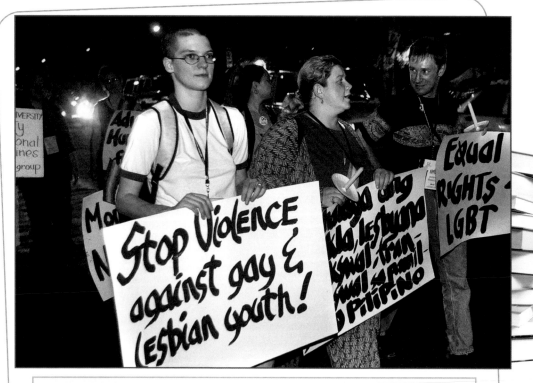

Even though transgenderism is more accepted now than ever, members of the LGBT community must continue to fight for equality and against discrimination.

harassment. Since the law also prohibits discrimination against transgender students, schools have no legal basis to deny students the right to wear the clothes they want or to be called by the name they want to be called by. Also, schools are required to provide access to bathrooms and locker rooms that respect transgender students' privacy and allow them to feel safe.

If a school does not do that on its own, it is necessary to point out the obligations to the school administration by making an official complaint to the principal. If the

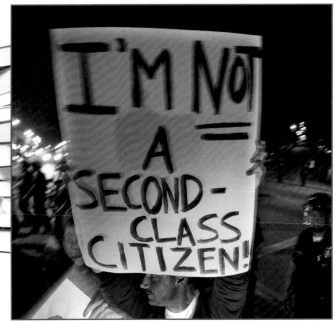

Even though there has been much progress in the acceptance of transgenderism, members of the LGBT community must continue to fight against discrimination.

complaint is in reply to a specific incident, that incident should be documented as thoroughly as possible, which includes asking witnesses to write down a description of what they observed. It is a good idea to present any complaint in written form and keep a copy to be able to document the complaint and ask for a particular solution. That way, you can follow up on the complaint and hold the person accepting the complaint accountable.

If the school's response is inadequate, it is possible to file a complaint with the school district. These dealings can take a lot of time to resolve, though. In the case of immediate danger, like experiencing violence or threats of violence, call the police and report the abuse to the school after you have found physical and emotional safety.

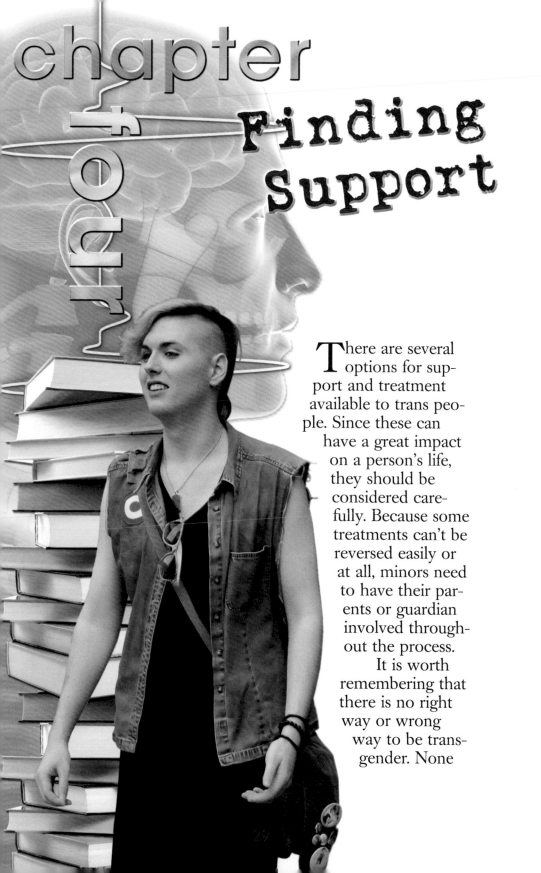

chapter four

Finding Support

There are several options for support and treatment available to trans people. Since these can have a great impact on a person's life, they should be considered carefully. Because some treatments can't be reversed easily or at all, minors need to have their parents or guardian involved throughout the process.

It is worth remembering that there is no right way or wrong way to be transgender. None of these options is something that you have to do. It all comes down to the individual, but often other factors (especially the high cost) come into play as well.

Mental Health

The official diagnostic book of the American Psychiatric Association (APA) lists gender identity disorder (GID), also called gender dysphoria, as a mental health condition. This is extremely controversial, as some people would rather see it classified as a medical condition and others

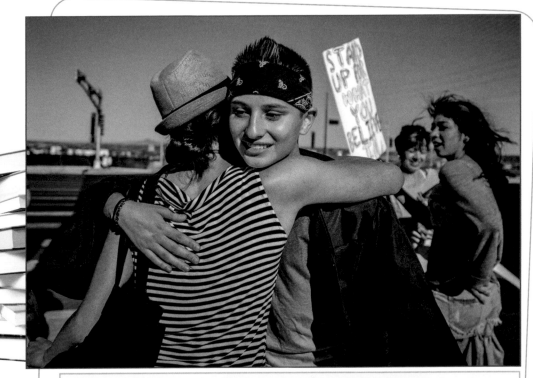

Support from peers is among the best ways to discover one's sexual identity. Damian Garcia, born a girl but who considers herself a boy, gets a hug of support after she fought to wear a male uniform to her graduation.

want to remove altogether the stigma of transgenderism being some kind of illness.

In the pamphlet "Answers to Your Questions About Transgender People, Gender Identity, and Gender Expression" available on its Web site, the APA explains that a "psychological state is considered a mental disorder only if it causes significant distress or disability. Many transgender people do not experience their gender as distressing or disabling, which implies that identifying as transgender does not constitute a mental disorder. For these individuals, the significant problem is finding affordable resources, such as counseling, hormone therapy, medical procedures, and the social support necessary to freely express their gender identity and minimize discrimination." Being diagnosed with GID can help in finding resources (e.g., when dealing with insurance companies), so there is a positive side to it. A note from a doctor can also go a long way when dealing with school officials and others. In addition, being diagnosed with GID is often a prerequisite for hormonal treatment and gender-affirming surgeries.

While being transgender does not mean a person is mentally ill, many trans people suffer from anxiety or depression as a result of the lack of acceptance in society and the discrimination they may experience. Psychotherapy may be needed to deal with those issues.

One thing to be wary of is so-called reparative therapy, which is often religiously motivated and aims to "cure" trans people. Since transgenderism is not an illness, there is nothing to cure, and reparative therapy is considered by many to be nothing but psychological abuse. It may lead the treated person to suppress who he or she is for a time, but it will not contribute to the person's well-being.

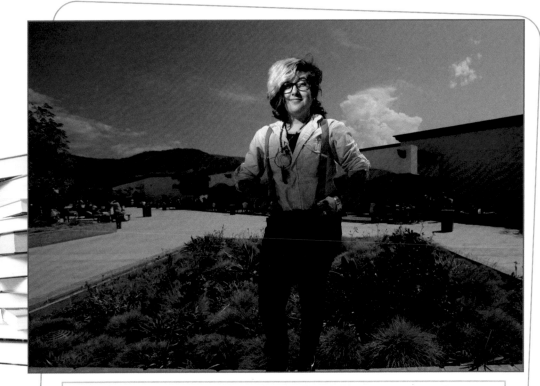

Adolescence can be a trying time for transgender youth but transgender student Benji Delgadillo took the fight for equality into the classroom by convincing his teacher to include members of the LGBT community in history lessons.

Transitioning

Some transgender people strive to permanently lead their life as the gender that they identify with. Transitioning from one gender to another can be done in several different ways, and not all transgender people interested in transitioning will go through the same process, either because they do not want to or because the options for medical and surgical treatment are too expensive.

Social Transition

Socially, transitioning starts with coming out, but it encompasses more than that. For the transperson transitioning socially, it is a learning experience to live in the world as their true self. Even if it goes unnoticed that they are transgender, many will find that they are treated differently because of the gender they now present themselves as versus what they were before. Men and women are still treated differently in society, and that might come as a bit of a shock to experience firsthand.

Hormonal Transition

Hormones are chemicals that convey messages within an organism to affect the development of cells. Sex hormones affect the development of the gonads and sexual characteristics. There are two main classes of sex hormones: androgens, which have a virilizing effect and, therefore, are often called male sex hormones; and estrogens, which are female sex hormones. (They are not really sex-specific hormones, as men also have estrogens and women have androgens, but not at the same level.) Taking synthetic hormones has a great impact on physical appearance and affects the emotional state of a person.

Since testosterone, the main male sex hormone, is very powerful, transwomen have to take androgen suppressants to reign in its effects as well as take female hormones. These female hormones bring about several changes, including an increase in breast tissue, softer skin texture, less body hair growth, and a decrease in muscle mass.

Transmen going through hormonal transition do not need to take any suppressants, just male hormones. These will cause menstruation to cease, body and facial hair growth to increase, and the voice to lower. They will also make it easier to increase muscle mass.

Transpeople undergoing hormone therapy will likely find that it has an impact on their emotions. For transmen, it may be more difficult to express emotion, while transwomen may find it easier than before.

Some effects of hormonal treatment are reversible if stopped, but others are not. It can have a negative impact on fertility, which is something that needs to be considered before hormonal transition is started.

While the effects of hormonal treatment can be severe, there are some things it will not change, like the voice of a transwoman who has been through puberty, which is why many choose to take voice lessons. Some physical aspects can only be changed through surgery.

Surgical Transition

These surgeries are commonly known as "sex change" or "sex reassignment" surgery, but because of the distinction between sex and gender, a better name would be gender-affirming surgery.

They tend to be extremely expensive because they are only rarely covered by insurance and usually have to be paid out of pocket. Therefore, many transgender people can't afford these surgeries or not as many as they would like, while others choose not to have them for reasons other than the cost.

One common type of surgery is chest surgery. While transwomen may experience breast growth caused by hormonal treatment, this will usually not reach the extent of that of a physically female person, so many will consider breast augmentation surgery as an option. Transwomen, on the other hand, will not experience a reduction of their breast tissue due to hormonal treatment. Depending on size, binding the breasts may be an option to hide them,

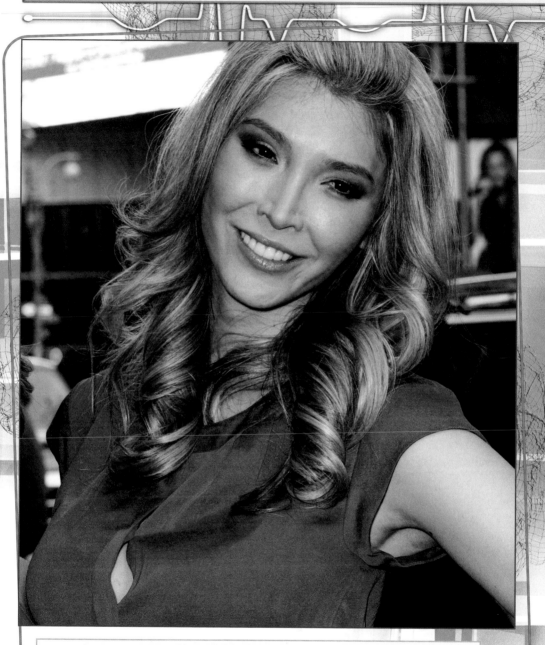

Transwoman Jenna Talackova, who began her transition as a teenager, competed in the Miss Universe Canada pageant after successfully fighting those who wanted to disqualify her for her transgenderism.

but that can lead to back pains and breathing difficulties. There are different surgical procedures to reconstruct the chest to look like that of a physically male person.

Genital surgery aims to remove the external reproductive organs that the person undergoing surgery was born with and to create those corresponding to the gender they identify with. This usually leads to better results for transwomen than for transmen, although some transmen are happy with the results and progress is still being made. It should be noted that the reproductive organs will not be fully functional after surgery. A transman will not be able

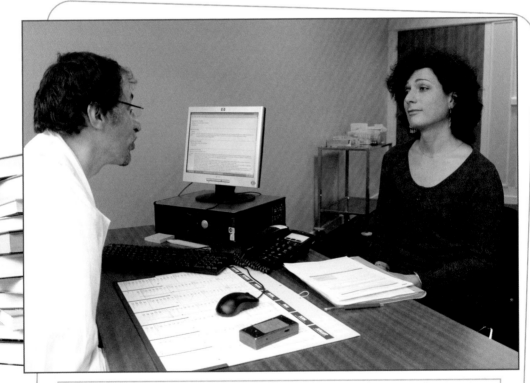

There are different medical options for trans people seeking to transition hormonally and/or surgically, which need to be discussed with a professional.

to father a child, and a transwoman will not be able to bear a child. Some transmen may opt to have their ovaries and/or uterus removed to avoid complications. Many transwomen have surgery on their face to make them look more feminine (e.g., a reshaping of the nose or jaw) or have their Adam's apple reduced.

Delaying Puberty

The changes brought on by puberty can be traumatic for transgender children. As their body reaches adulthood, the discrepancy between their gender identity and their biological sex becomes more apparent. It is possible to delay puberty through the use of drugs called GnRH inhibitors, which shut down the typical hormonal surges and, as a result, prevent permanent changes in a child's body–for several years, if need be. This gives the family time until the transgender child comes to a decision on whether he or she wants to undergo hormonal or surgical transition. If the medicine is discontinued, puberty will start normally after some time without any negative effect due to the delay.

The positive effect for young trans people whose puberty is delayed through GnRH inhibitors is that future surgeries are less likely to be necessary because their bodies do not go through the changes that they may want to reverse later. This is especially true for transgirls, who will not develop an Adam's apple, typically male facial features, body and facial hair, and a lower voice.

A transgirl using GnRH inhibitors and estrogens will go through female puberty, and a transboy using the inhibitors and androgens will go through male puberty with all the physical and emotional changes it usually entails. These changes will be more drastic than those

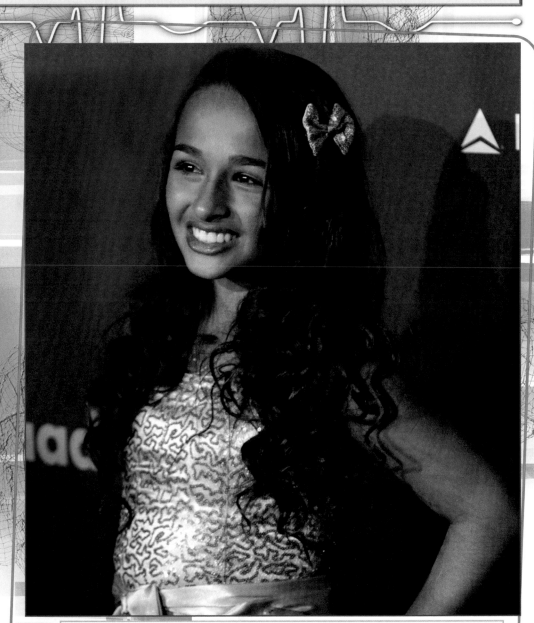

Transgender teen Jazz Jennings arrives at the GLAAD (Gay & Lesbian Alliance Against Defamation) Media Awards in Los Angeles, California. Finding support from groups such as GLAAD is important for young people when discovering their gender identity.

experienced by trans people undergoing hormonal transition after they went through puberty. However, they will not alter the reproductive organs, which can only be changed surgically.

One thing to consider is that a transgender child using GnRH inhibitors and hormones will not be fertile. For the male body to produce sperm, it has to go through male puberty, and for the female body's eggs to mature, it has to go through female puberty. There is a slight chance that fertility can be achieved if the treatment is stopped for a lengthy amount of time and the person goes through the puberty corresponding to his or her birth sex. But there is no guarantee that it will work, and complications are likely. Even if this choice should mean to give up one's fertility, there are other ways to start a family.

anatomical sex The physical structure of one's body that makes it male or female, based on chromosomes, gonads, hormones, and the internal and external reproductive organs.

coming out Short for "coming out of the closet," the act of disclosing one's sexual orientation.

cross-dresser A person who likes wearing clothes that are associated with the opposite sex.

FtM (female-to-male) A person who was born anatomically female but identifies as male; also called a transman (or transboy, depending on age).

gender A social construct of what is typically associated with one sex.

gender expression The way a person externally communicates his or her gender identity (clothes, haircut, mannerisms, etc.).

gender identity A person's innermost concept of which gender he or she belongs to.

gender role What is traditionally expected of and considered appropriate for a male or female in society.

genderqueer People who feel they are neither male nor female, but rather a mix of the two or maybe something different altogether.

intersex A person born with anatomical characteristics that are neither 100 percent male nor 100 percent female.

MtF (male-to-female) A person who was born anatomically male but identifies as female; also called a transwoman (or transgirl, depending on age).

sexual orientation Whom one is romantically and sexually attracted to. Contrary to popular belief, not all transgender people are homosexual.

transgender Anyone whose behaviour does not match traditional gender norms.

transition The process through which a transgender person tries to reach a gender expression that matches his or her gender identity more closely.

transsexual Someone whose gender identity does not match the sex that he or she was assigned at birth.

Canadian Professional Association for Transgender Health
(CPATH)
201-1770 Fort Street
Victoria, BC V8R 1J5
Canada
(250) 592-6183
Web site: http://www.cpath.ca
The largest national professional organization for transgender health in the world is devoted to furthering the understanding and health care of those with gender variant identities.

Gender Spectrum
539 Glen Drive
San Leandro, CA 94577
(520) 567-3977
Web site: http://www.genderspectrum.org
Gender Spectrum offers consultation, training, and events in order to create a gender-sensitive environment for children and teens.

Human Rights Campaign (HRC)
1640 Rhode Island Avenue NW
Washington, DC 20036-3278
(202) 216-1572
Web site: http://www.hrc.org
With more than 1.5 million members, the HRC is the largest civil rights organization working to achieve equality for lesbian, gay, bisexual, and transgender Americans.

Parents, Families and Friends of Lesbians and Gays (PFLAG)
PFLAG National Office
1828 L Street NW, Suite 660
Washington, DC 20036
(202) 467-8180
Web site: http://www.pflag.org
Through more than 350 chapters across the United States, PFLAG provides education, advocacy, and support to promote the health and well-being of lesbian, gay, bisexual, and transgender persons and their families and friends.

Trans Youth Equality Foundation
1 Forest Avenue
Portland, ME 04101
(207) 478-4087
Web site: http://www.transyouthequality.org
The Trans Youth Equality Foundation focuses on providing education and support for transgender children and their families.

Web Sites

Due to the changing nature of Internet links, Rosen Publishing has developed an online list of Web sites related to the subject of this book. This site is updated regularly. Please use this link to access the list:

http://www.rosenlinks.com/TMH/Gend

Beam, Cris. *Transparent: Love, Family, and Living the T with Transgender Teenagers*. Orlando, FL: Mariner Books, 2008.

Beemyn, Genny, and Susan Rankin. *The Lives of Transgender People*. New York, NY: Columbia University Press, 2011.

Biegel, Stuart. *The Right to Be Out: Sexual Orientation and Gender Identity in America's Public Schools*. Minneapolis, MN: University of Minneapolis Press, 2010.

Butch, Brian, and Rebecca Haskell. *Get That Freak: Homophobia and Transphobia in High Schools*. Halifax, Canada: Fernwood Publishing, 2010.

Cahill, Sean, and Jason Cianciotto. *LGBT Youth in America's Schools*. Ann Arbor, MI: University of Michigan Press, 2012.

DeWitt, Peter. *Dignity for All: Safeguarding LGBT Students*. Thousand Oaks, CA: Corwin Press, 2012.

Driver, Susan. *Queer Youth Cultures*. Albany, NY: State University of New York Press, 2008.

Duncan, Neil, and Ian Rivers, eds. *Bullying. Experiences and Discourses of Sexuality and Gender*. New York, NY: Routledge, 2012.

Giordano, Simona. *Children with Gender Identity Disorder: A Clinical, Ethical, and Legal Analysis*. New York, NY: Routledge, 2013.

Herman, Joanne. *Transgender Explained for Those Who Are Not*. Bloomington, IN: AuthorHouse, 2009.

Huegel, Kelly. *GLBTQ: The Survival Guide for Gay, Lesbian, Bisexual, Transgender, and Questioning Teens*. Minneapolis, MN: Free Spirit Publishing, 2011.

Krieger, Irwin. *Helping Your Transgender Teen: A Guide for Parents*. New Haven, CT: Genderwise Press, 2011.

Miller, Terry, and Dan Savage. *It Gets Better: Coming Out, Overcoming Bullying, and Creating a Life Worth Living*. New York, NY: Dutton, 2011.

Nadal, Kevin L. *That's So Gay!: Microaggressions and the Lesbian, Gay, Bisexual, and Transgender Community*. Washington, DC: American PsychologicalAssociation, 2013.

Seba, Jaime. *Feeling Wrong in Your Own Body: Understanding What It Means to Be Transgender*. Broomall, PA: Mason Crest Publishing, 2011.

Stewart, Chuck, ed. *The Greenwood Encyclopedia of LGBT Issues Worldwide*. Santa Barbara, CA: Greenwood Press, 2010.

Strauss, Susan. *Sexual Harassment and Bullying: A Guide to Keeping Kids Safe and Holding Schools Accountable*. Lanham, MD: Rowman & Littlefield Publishers, 2012.

Stryker, Susan. *Transgender History*. Berkeley, CA: Seal Press, 2008.

Webber, Carlisle K. *Gay, Lesbian, Bisexual, Transgender and Questioning Teen Literature: A Guide to Reading Interests*. Santa Barbara, CA: Libraries Unlimited, 2010.

Index

About the Author

Nicki Peter Petrikowski is a literary scholar, as well as an editor, author, and translator. Out of respect for several of his friends in particular, and the idea of equality and human rights in general, he supports the LGBT social movement.

Photo Credits

Cover (right, inset left center, bottom), pp. 1 (inset center, bottom, 12, 21, 23, 24, 32 © AP Images; cover and p. 1 (top left inset), p. 20 Ariwasabi/Shutterstock.com; cover, pp. 1, 3 (head and brain illustration) © iStockphoto.com/Yakobchuk: p. 3 (laptop) © iStockphoto.com/Colonel; pp. 4, 12, 20, 29 (head and brain illustration) © iStockphoto.com/angelhell; p. 4 mihailomilovanovic/Shutterstock.com; p. 5 Roderick Chen/First Light/Getty Images; pp. 7, 19, iStockphoto/Thinkstock; p. 8 James Siedl/Shutterstock.com; p. 10 Matt Jelonek/WireImage/Getty Images; p. 14 Stephane Bidouze/Shutterstock.com; p. 16 Michael Tran/FilmMagic/Getty Images; p. 17 maturos1812/Shutterstock.com. 27 Joel Nito/AFP/Getty Images; p. 28 David McNew/Getty Images; p. 29 rmnoa357/Shutterstock; p. 30 Roberto E. Rosales/ Albuquerque Journal/ZUMA Press ; p. 32 Margot Petrowski/Shutterstock.com; p. 35 Ray Tamarra/Getty Images; p. 36 BSIP/Universal Images Group/Getty Images; p. 38 Jonathan Alcorn/Reuters/Landov; multiple interior pages (books) © iStockphoto.com/zoomstudio.

Designer: Nelson Sá; Editor: Nicholas Croce;
Photo Researcher: Marty Levick